MUDRAS FOR TEACHERS

Enhance Voice Clarity, Cultivate Emotional Resilience, Boost Classroom Presence, and Empower Teaching With Hand Gestures

By

SHILPA MEHTA

PREFACE

Namaste!

Writing *"Mudras for Teachers: Enhance Voice Clarity, Cultivate Emotional Resilience, Boost Classroom Presence, and Empower Teaching With Hand Gestures"* has been a deeply personal journey for me. As an educator, I have always sought ways to enrich my teaching practice and improve my own well-being. The challenges of managing a classroom, meeting academic standards, and maintaining personal balance have driven me to explore various tools and techniques that support both my professional and personal growth.

As a yoga teacher, my journey into whole-body mudras and meditation began many years ago. However, it was my encounter with Hasta mudras through a dedicated yoga practitioner that truly inspired me. Witnessing their transformative impact, I felt compelled to share these powerful practices with fellow educators, believing they too could benefit immensely.

This book is the culmination of three decades of my experience and research into how mudras can benefit teachers. It is designed not only to introduce you to these powerful hand gestures but also to provide practical guidance on integrating them into your daily routine. The techniques presented here are those I have found to be most beneficial in my own teaching practice and personal life.

"May these practices benefit all educators as much as they have benefited me. This book is a heartfelt gift to the entire educator community."

Warm regards,

Shilpa Mehta

DEDICATION

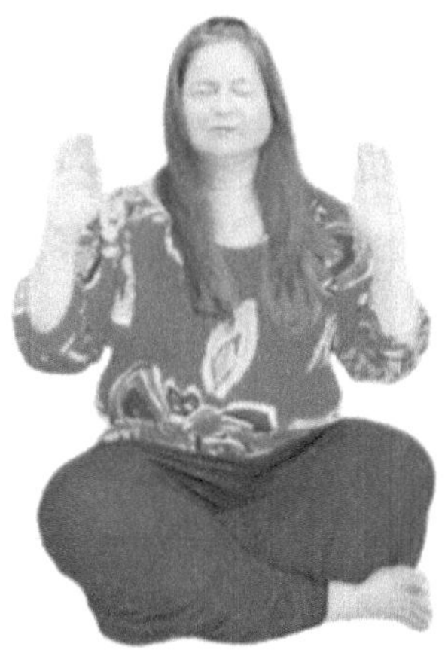

To all educators who ignite minds and nurture hearts—your dedication is the essence of teaching.

To my mentors and colleagues, whose wisdom and support have guided me.

To my students, past and present, whose enthusiasm inspires me daily.

To my daughter Reekta, son-in-law Karan, and grandchildren, whose love and faith in me have been a constant source of strength and joy.

To my sister Trupti, Dr. Rohit Gandhi, and my friend Dr. Sanjivv Gandhi, whose unwavering love and encouragement have been invaluable.

This book is my humble offering to my late mother and Yogi Vinod, whose influence and guidance continue to inspire me.

Your support has made this work possible, and your spirit shines through every page.

Thank you for being a part of this journey and for helping to make this dream a reality.

Why Is This Book For You

Teaching is a rewarding but demanding job that requires physical, emotional, and mental resilience. This book offers practical tools for teachers to manage stress, improve vocal health, enhance hearing, support heart health, maintain good posture, and achieve relaxation.

By integrating these practices into your daily routine, you can cultivate calm, focus, and resilience, benefiting both yourself and your students. The mudras and meditation techniques are simple, effective, and easy to fit into a busy schedule.

"Mudras for Educators" provides clear instructions and real-life applications to help you enhance your well-being and create a supportive, mindful classroom environment. Discover how these ancient practices can transform your teaching experience and lead to a healthier, happier, and more balanced life.

Table Of Contents

Chapter 1: Understanding Mudras

What are Mudras?

Mudras are ancient hand gestures used in yoga, meditation, and spiritual practices. These symbolic gestures, often performed with the hands and fingers, are powerful tools for channelling energy and enhancing physical, mental, and spiritual well-being. The term "mudra" means "seal" or "sign," and each gesture creates a subtle connection between different parts of the body, mind, and consciousness.

Types of Mudras

- Hand Mudras (Hasta Mudras): These are the most common and widely practiced mudras, involving specific positioning of the fingers and hands. Each hand mudra represents different aspects of life, emotions, and energies. For example, Gyan Mudra.

- Body Mudras (Kaya Mudras): These mudras involve specific body postures or movements that aid in directing energy flow within the body. Like Viparita Karni.

- Lock Mudras (Bandha Mudras): These mudras involve muscular contractions and body locks that regulate the flow of energy, particularly in Kundalini yoga practices. Mula Bandha, for instance.

Mudras and Elements

Our Body is made of five elements, viz., Earth (Prithvi), Water (Jal), Fire (Agni), Air (Vayu) and Ether (Akash).

Each finger in hand mudras is associated with one of the five elements:

- Thumb: Fire element (Agni)

- Index finger: Air element (Vayu)

- Middle finger: Ether or space element (Akasha)

- Ring finger: Earth element (Prithvi)

- Little finger: Water element (Jala)

The five fingers of our hand when joined in specific manner enable us to achieve the balance and harmony of these vital elements.

(Kindly check the picture in the next page.)

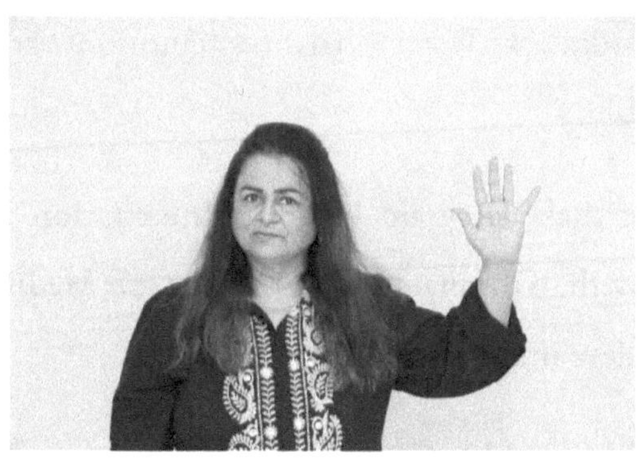

How Mudras Work

Mudras operate on the principle that the human body is a complex network of energy channels (nadis) through which life force energy (Prana) flows. By forming specific gestures or postures, mudras facilitate the redirection and enhancement of this Pranic energy. This alignment of energy is believed to harmonize the physical, mental, and spiritual dimensions of an individual, promoting holistic well-being.

Benefits of Mudras

- Physical: They improve blood circulation, enhance finger flexibility, and relieve muscle tension. For instance, Prithvi Mudra (Mudra of Earth) helps combat physical fatigue.

- Mental and Emotional: Mudras can calm the mind, reduce stress, and boost mental clarity. Varuna Mudra

(Mudra of Water) balances emotions and promotes stability.

- Spiritual: They aid in deeper meditation and spiritual growth. Dhyana Mudra (Mudra of Meditation) helps achieve inner tranquility and focus.

Practical Considerations

Choosing the Right Mudra: Select mudras based on your needs, such as improving concentration, reducing stress, or promoting relaxation. Tailor them to address specific challenges and classroom dynamics.

Safety and Precautions: Mudras are generally safe, but individuals with medical conditions or physical limitations should consult a healthcare professional before practicing advanced mudras or extended sessions.

Key Tips for Effective Mudra Practice

Mudras can be practiced while seated, lying down, standing, or walking. Ensure your posture is symmetrical and centered, and stay focused and relaxed.

- Seated: Keep your back straight, feet firmly on the floor. If on a cushion, sit upright with both knees at the same height, supported by a cushion if needed. Hands rest on thighs, shoulders relaxed, chest open, chin gently pulled back, neck long and relaxed.

- Lying down: Rest on your back, with a small pillow under your head and a cushion under your knees for support.

- Standing: Keep legs shoulder-width apart, knees relaxed, and toes pointing forward.

- Walking: Move in an even, calm, and rhythmic manner.

For longer sessions, seated meditation is ideal. Breathe evenly, slowly, and gently. End meditation gradually, stretching your arms and legs.

Comfort and relaxation are essential to avoid tension and ensure smooth energy flow during mudra practice.

Importance of Breath Control in Mudra

While forming a mudra, slow your breathing to make it deep, rhythmic, and flowing. This helps reduce thoughts and calms the mind. The effect of the mudra intensifies when combined with a meditative posture, hand focus, and breath observation.

Watching your natural breath flow or consciously directing it enhances the mudra's impact. Using visualizations and affirmations can prevent the practice from becoming routine and deepen the effects.

Performing Hast Mudras with both hands is more effective than using one hand.

Science Behind Mudras

Scientific studies in recent times have examined the physiological and neurological mechanisms related to mudras. Research show that specific mudras can stimulate corresponding brain regions, influencing neural pathways and neurotransmitter activity. These effects enhance cognitive functions, reduce stress, and promote overall well-being.

Conclusion

Understanding the basic aspects of different types of mudras, with their elemental associations, and therapeutic benefits, prepares us to explore their practical applications in everyday life and specific contexts like education.

In the following chapters, we will delve deeper into mudras particularly beneficial for educators, providing techniques and insights to enhance teaching effectiveness and personal well-being.

Chapter 2: Stress Management

Stress In Teaching: Understanding The Causes

Teachers worldwide face significant stress and burnout be it in Government or Private School, impacting their health and well-being. Here are key reasons:

Challenges Faced by Teachers

- Managing lesson plans, grading, and administrative tasks leads to long hours and little personal time.

- Large class sizes especially in government schools, making it difficult to give individual attention and manage behaviour.

- Excessive paperwork and meetings reduce teaching time, adding stress.

- Focus on standardized test performance can increase pressure.

- Insufficient materials and infrastructure, especially in government schools.

- Providing emotional support and managing behavioural issues.

- Uncertainty about job stability, particularly in private schools, adds stress.

- Balancing high expectations from parents with students' needs can be overwhelming.

Examples of Stress in Teaching

1. Mrs. Sharma in a Government School: Mrs. Sharma teaches a large class of 55 students with limited resources. She often works late to prepare lesson plans and create materials, which affects her health and well-being.

2. Mrs. Verma in a Private School: Mrs. Verma faces high pressure to maintain academic standards. She spends extra hours grading and attending meetings, and constant scrutiny from parents and management increases her stress.

Teachers experience significant stress due to their demanding roles, leading to anxiety, depression, poor coping skills, and unhealthy behaviours like overeating. Chronic stress increases the risk of burnout, mental health issues, and physical ailments like fatigue and headaches. Finding healthier coping strategies is crucial for teachers' well-being and effectiveness both at work and at home.

"Healthy teachers create healthy classrooms. Your wellness matters!"

This book is your guide to positive health. Start with simple movements and mudras, which can help alleviate stress, anxiety, and depression, especially when combined with pranayama. Let's begin this transformative journey together, focusing on both preventive and curative measures for a fulfilling teaching career.

1. Anjali Mudra (Gesture of Reverence)

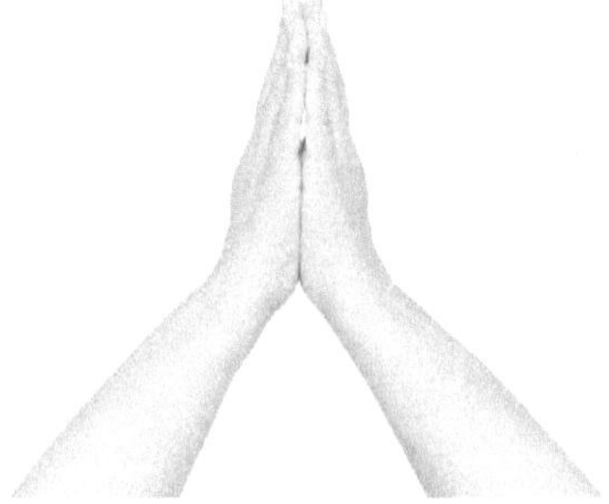

Anjali, Atmanjali or Namaste Mudra, is known as the Gesture of Reverence or Prayer Pose. It is a simple yet profound mudra used in yoga and meditation. It involves pressing the palms together in front of the heart, symbolizing respect, gratitude, and balance.

Forming the Mudra:

- Sit or stand comfortably with your back straight and shoulders relaxed.

- Place your hands in front of your chest with the palms pressed together.

- Bring the palms of your hands together at the center of your chest.

- Keep the fingers pointing upwards and the thumbs gently touching your sternum.

Breathing:

- Take a deep, calming breath in through your nose.

- Exhale slowly and evenly, maintaining a sense of centeredness and balance.

- Maintain a steady and rhythmic breathing pattern throughout the practice.

Benefits:

- Centres the mind, improving concentration and mental clarity.

- Induces a sense of inner peace and reduces stress.

- Encourages feelings of gratitude and reverence.

- Supports emotional and mental balance, aiding in overall well-being.

Applications for Teachers:

- Integrate Anjali Mudra into your daily routine to cultivate calmness and balance.

- Use this mudra before starting your classes to centre yourself and set a positive tone.

- Practice Anjali Mudra during short breaks to alleviate stress and regain focus.

By regularly practicing Anjali Mudra, teachers can experience enhanced focus, reduced stress, and a greater sense of balance, contributing to a more harmonious and effective teaching environment.

2. Abhaya Mudra (Gesture of Fearlessness)

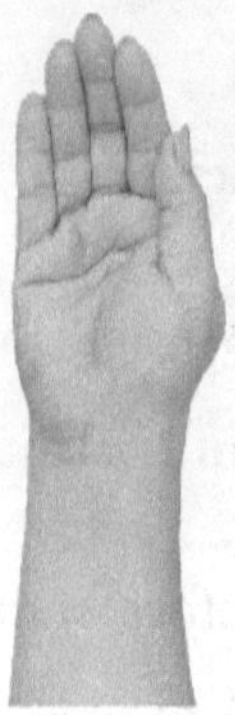

Abhaya Mudra, also known as the Gesture of Fearlessness, is a symbolic hand gesture that represents protection, courage, and reassurance. The gesture involves raising the right hand with the palm facing outward, symbolizing a promise of safety and a call to face challenges with confidence.

Forming the Mudra:

- Sit comfortably with your back straight and shoulders relaxed.

- Raise your right hand to shoulder height, with the palm facing outward.

- Keep the fingers extended and the thumb relaxed.

- Your left hand can rest on your lap or in a relaxed position.

Breathing:

- Inhale deeply through your nose, drawing in a sense of strength and reassurance.

- Exhale slowly and evenly, allowing any tension or fear to dissolve.

Benefits:

- Fosters a sense of inner courage and confidence, empowering you to face challenges with calm.

- Alleviates anxiety and promote a sense of safety and protection.

- Strengthens your resolve and supports emotional resilience.

- Creates a nurturing and supportive environment in the classroom.

Applications for Teachers:

- Incorporate Abhaya Mudra into your daily routine to build inner strength and resilience.

- Use this mudra before or during classes to instill confidence and a sense of security.

- Practice Abhaya Mudra during stressful moments to reduce anxiety and regain composure.

By integrating Abhaya Mudra into your daily practice, teachers can cultivate greater confidence, reduce anxiety, and foster a supportive teaching environment, enhancing their overall effectiveness and well-being.

3. Prana Mudra (Gesture of Vitality)

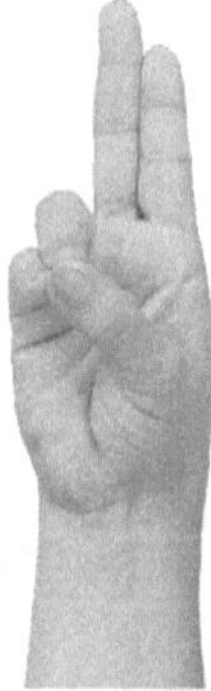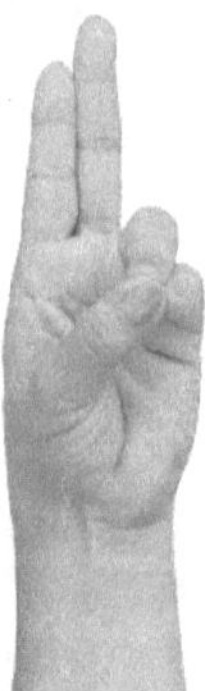

Introduction:

Prana Mudra, known as the Gesture of Vitality, is a hand gesture used to enhance life energy and promote overall vitality. This mudra involves touching the tips of the ring and little fingers to the tip of the thumb, while keeping the other fingers extended.

Forming the Mudra:

- Sit comfortably with your back straight and shoulders relaxed.

- Place your hands on your knees with your palms facing upwards.

- Touch the tips of your ring and little fingers to the tip of your thumb.

- Keep the index and middle fingers extended.

Breathing:

- Inhale deeply through your nose, feeling the breath energize your body.

- Exhale slowly and completely through your nose, releasing any tension or fatigue.

- Maintain a steady and rhythmic breathing pattern throughout the practice.

Benefits:

- Invigorates the body and mind, increasing overall energy and vitality.

- Alleviates feelings of tiredness and exhaustion, revitalizing your spirit.

- Promotes a sense of physical and mental well-being, supporting overall health.

- Balances and harmonizes the body's energy flow, enhancing overall vitality.

Applications for Teachers:

- Integrate Prana Mudra into your daily routine to boost energy levels and combat fatigue.

- Use this mudra before starting your classes to increase your energy and focus for a productive day.

- Practice Prana Mudra during breaks to rejuvenate and maintain high energy levels throughout the day.

- Employ this mudra to reduce stress and enhance overall vitality during demanding times.

By regularly practicing Prana Mudra, teachers can experience increased energy, reduced fatigue, and a greater sense of overall well-being, contributing to a more dynamic and effective teaching experience.

4. Kaleshwar Mudra (Gesture of Divine Protection)

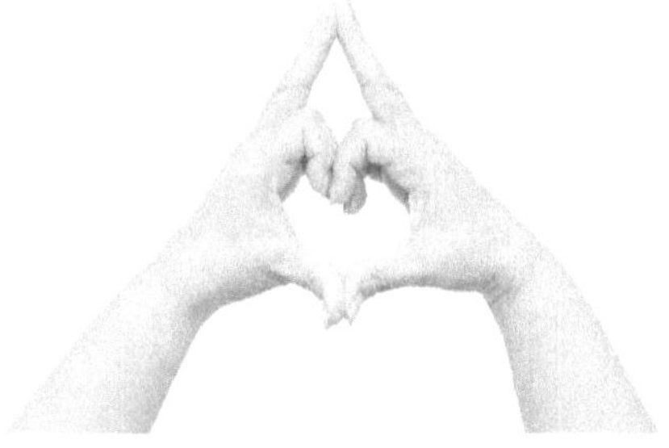

Kaleshwar Mudra, often referred to as the Gesture of Divine Protection, is a hand gesture used in yoga and meditation to cultivate inner strength, peace, and protection. This mudra involves positioning the hands in a specific way to channel energy and create a sense of sacredness and stability.

Forming the Mudra:

- Sit comfortably with your back straight and shoulders relaxed.

- Bring your hands together in front of your chest, with the palms facing each other and fingers pointing upward.

- Interlace your fingers so that the tips of your index fingers and thumbs touch, forming a small diamond shape.

- Keep the other fingers extended, creating a gentle, protective frame around your heart area.

Breathing:

- Inhale deeply through your nose, feeling a sense of expansion and stability in your chest.

- Exhale slowly and evenly through your nose, releasing any tension and cultivating inner peace.

- Maintain a calm and rhythmic breathing pattern throughout the practice.

Benefits:

- Builds inner resilience and strength, allowing you to face challenges with confidence.

- Promotes emotional stability and tranquility, reducing stress and anxiety.

- Supports mental focus and clarity, aiding in better decision-making and concentration.

- Creates a feeling of sacredness and protection, reinforcing a sense of security and well-being.

Applications for Teachers:

- Incorporate into your daily routine to cultivate inner strength and emotional balance.

- Use before starting your classes to center yourself and create a sense of calm and protection.

- Practice during stressful moments to restore emotional equilibrium and enhance mental clarity.

- Include this gesture in your mindfulness or meditation sessions to reinforce a sense of inner peace and security.

By regularly practicing Kaleshwar Mudra, teachers can experience enhanced inner strength, emotional balance, and a greater sense of protection, contributing to a more harmonious and focused teaching environment.

5. Guided meditation for relaxation.

This time is for you to unwind and reconnect with a sense of calm. Let's begin.

Settling In:

- Take a comfortable chair, and settle in.

- Sit with your back straight and shoulders relaxed. Place your feet flat on the floor and rest your hands gently on the arm rests or in your lap.

- Close your eyes if you feel comfortable doing so, or keep them softly focused on a point in front of you.

Deep Breathing:

- Take a deep breath in through your nose, feeling your abdomen expand fully.

- Hold the breath for a moment, then exhale slowly through your mouth, releasing any tension.

- Continue this deep, slow breathing, inhaling deeply and exhaling completely for 5 times.

- With each breath, imagine inhaling calmness and exhaling stress.

Visualization:

- Imagine a warm, soothing light at the top of your head. This light is gentle and calming, spreading warmth and relaxation throughout your body.

- Visualize this light slowly descending, enveloping your entire body in its warmth. As it moves down, it melts away any stress or tension you may be holding.

- Feel the warmth reaching your feet, grounding you in a deep sense of relaxation and peace.

Affirmations:

Silently or aloud, repeat these affirmations to yourself:

- "I am calm and at peace."

- "I release all tension and stress."

Reconnecting:

- Gradually bring your awareness back to the present moment. Notice the sensations of your body in the chair, the sounds around you, and the feeling of your breath.

- When you feel ready, gently wiggle your fingers and toes, bringing movement back into your body.

- Open your eyes slowly if they were closed, and take a moment to notice how you feel.

Ending:

- Before concluding, take a deep breath in, and as you exhale, let go of any remaining tension.

- When you're ready, move your body gently.

Carry this sense of relaxation you've cultivated during this meditation *as you continue with your day.*

Conclusion

Incorporating stress management mudras like Anjali, Abhay, Prana, and Kaleshwar into your daily routine can significantly enhance relaxation and overall well-being. These mudras, along with guided meditation for relaxation, offer powerful tools to alleviate stress and promote mental clarity. By practicing these techniques regularly, educators can cultivate a calm and centered mindset, improving both personal wellness and teaching effectiveness.

Chapter 3: Importance of Correct Posture

Importance of Posture

- Prevents musculoskeletal disorders by reducing strain on muscles, ligaments, and joints.

- Supports spinal health, lowering the risk of back and neck pain.

- Improves breathing and circulation by allowing full lung expansion and enhancing blood flow.

- Enhances energy levels through efficient muscle use.

- Boosts confidence and presence with positive body language.

- Facilitates better eye contact and communication with students.

- Promotes long-term mobility and health, aiding active aging and quality of life.

Good posture supports physical health and enhances teaching effectiveness and overall well-being.

Tips for Maintaining Proper Posture:

- Be mindful of your posture and adjust throughout the day.

- Use ergonomic furniture to support proper alignment.

- Take frequent breaks to stand, stretch, and move.

- Strengthen core muscles with exercises for better posture.

- Distribute weight evenly when standing, keep feet flat and back supported when sitting.

1. Merudanda Mudra (Spine Mudra)

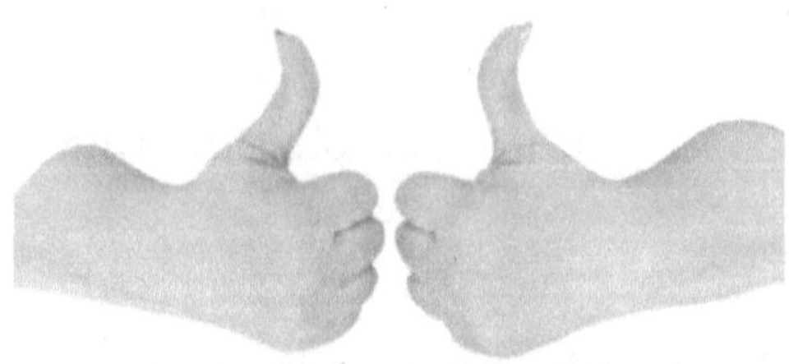

Meru' refers to the sacred mountain, and 'danda' means staff. Merudanda, the name of the spinal column, represents the central axis of energy in the body, balanced with stability and centeredness. It is also known as the Spine Mudra, and promotes the flow of energy along the spine, improving posture, and enhancing overall vitality.

Forming the Mudra:

- Sit in a comfortable position, either on a chair with your feet flat on the ground or on the floor in a cross-legged position.

- Keep your spine straight, shoulders relaxed, and hands resting on your knees or in your lap.

- Curl your fingers inward, leaving your thumbs extended.

- Point your thumbs upward for Merudanda Mudra.

Breathing:

- Inhale deeply through your nose, feeling the expansion in your chest and abdomen.

- Exhale slowly through your nose, maintaining the mudra and focusing on your central axis.

- Continue this rhythmic breathing for 5-10 minutes, or as long as you feel comfortable.

Benefits:

- Aligns the body's energy along the central axis, improving posture and stability.

- Balances and harmonizes the body's energy flow, fostering a sense of groundedness and stability.

- Maintains mental and physical balance, enhancing focus and concentration.

- Aligns the spine and improving overall posture, reducing physical strain.

Applications for Teachers:

- Integrate Merudanda Mudra into your daily routine to enhance posture and stability.

- Use it before classes to ground yourself and improve focus.

- Practice during short breaks to refresh your posture and balance.

- Include it in your daily practices to support spinal alignment and reduce strain from prolonged standing or sitting.

By incorporating Merudanda Mudra into your daily routine, you can enhance your posture, reduce back pain, and promote overall well-being, leading to a more effective and enjoyable teaching experience.

2. Vayu Mudra (Gesture of Air)

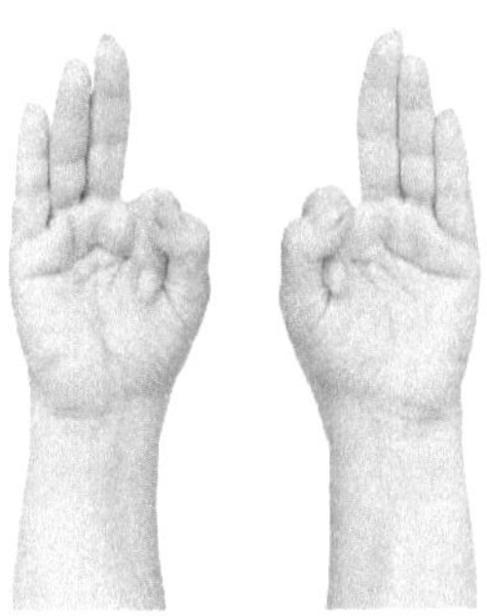

Introduction:

Vayu Mudra, also known as the Mudra of Air, is a hand gesture that helps balance the air element within the body. This mudra helps alleviate conditions related to air imbalances, such as joint pain, arthritis, and gas-related problems.

Forming the Mudra:

- Sit in a comfortable position, either on a chair with your feet flat on the ground or on the floor in a cross-legged position.

- Keep your spine straight, shoulders relaxed, and hands resting on your knees or in your lap.

- Bend your index finger and press it against the base of your thumb. Gently press the thumb on the bent index finger. Keep the other three fingers extended but relaxed.

Breathing:

- Inhale deeply through your nose, feeling the expansion in your chest and abdomen.

- Exhale slowly through your nose, releasing any tension while maintaining the mudra.

- Maintain a calm and rhythmic breathing pattern throughout the practice.

Benefits:

- Balances the air element in the body, reducing issues like bloating, gas, and joint pain.

- Relieves joint pain and stiffness, promoting better mobility.

- Enhances mental clarity and focus, aiding in better decision-making and concentration.

- Promotes a sense of calm and reduces stress and anxiety, fostering emotional stability.

Applications for Teachers:

- Incorporate Vayu Mudra into your daily routine to manage stress and maintain overall well-being.

- Use it before starting your classes to center yourself and enhance mental clarity.

- Practice it during stressful moments to restore emotional equilibrium and reduce anxiety.

- Include it in your mindfulness or meditation sessions to enhance focus and promote a sense of calm.

By regularly practicing Vayu Mudra, teachers can experience reduced stress, enhanced mental clarity, and relief from joint pain, contributing to a more effective and harmonious teaching environment.

3. Kati Mudra (Back Mudra)

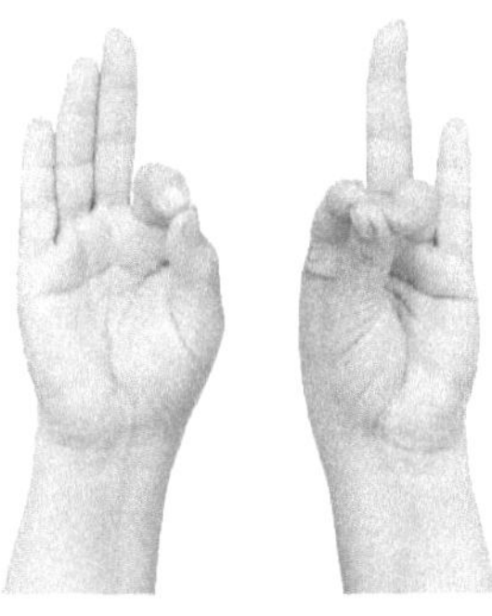

Introduction:

Kati Mudra, also known as Back Mudra, is a hand gesture designed to alleviate back pain. This mudra helps balance the body's energies and provides relief from both chronic and acute back discomfort, improving overall flexibility and strength.

Forming the Mudra:

- Right Hand:

  o Touch the tips of the thumb, middle finger, and little finger together.

  o Keep the index and ring fingers extended.

- Left Hand:

  o Touch the tip of the index finger to the base of the thumb.

  o Keep the other fingers extended.

Breathing:

- Inhale deeply through your nose, allowing your chest and abdomen to expand.

- Exhale slowly through your nose, releasing tension while maintaining the mudra.

- Maintain a calm and rhythmic breathing pattern throughout the practice.

Benefits:

- Relieves pain in the lower, middle, and upper back.

- Enhances flexibility and strength of the back.

- Prevents muscle tension and cramps.

- Improves the flow of prana and positive energy, removing negative energy.

- Balances the body's energy flow.

Applications for Teachers:

- Incorporate Kati Mudra into your daily routine to alleviate back pain caused by long hours of standing or sitting.

- Use it during breaks or at the end of the day to relax and relieve tension.

- Practice it lying down for lower back pain relief, ensuring your spine is comfortably supported.

- Include it in your mindfulness or meditation sessions to enhance overall well-being and maintain a neutral spine posture.

By regularly practicing Kati Mudra, teachers can experience reduced back pain, improved posture, and enhanced flexibility, contributing to a more comfortable and effective teaching environment.

4. Sitting Parvatasana (Seated Mountain Pose)

The human spine, or vertebral column, is a complex structure that provides support, protects the spinal cord. It allows for several types of movements:

- Forward

- Backward

- Upward

- Sideward

- Twisting

Sitting Parvatasana provides a complete range of spinal movements and can be effectively practiced on a chair.

Steps:

- Choose a sturdy chair without wheels, or position your chair against a wall for stability.

- Sit comfortably with your feet flat on the floor.

- Push your buttocks towards the backrest for support.

- Place your arms by your sides, palms facing upward.

- Raise your arms above your head, joining your palms in Namaste.

Forward Bend:

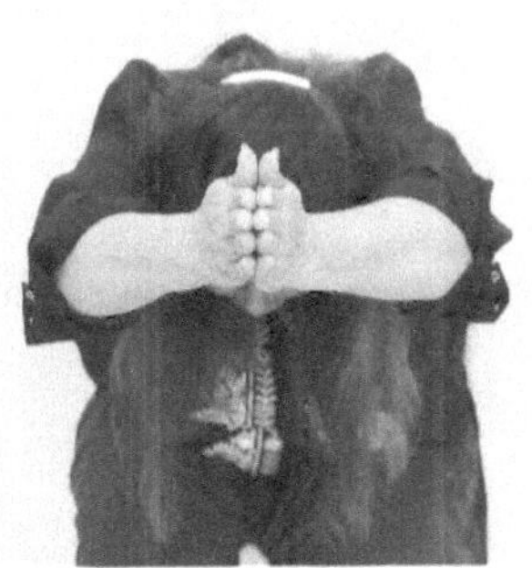

Keep your elbows straight and bend forward, maintaining the Namaste position.

Backward Stretch:

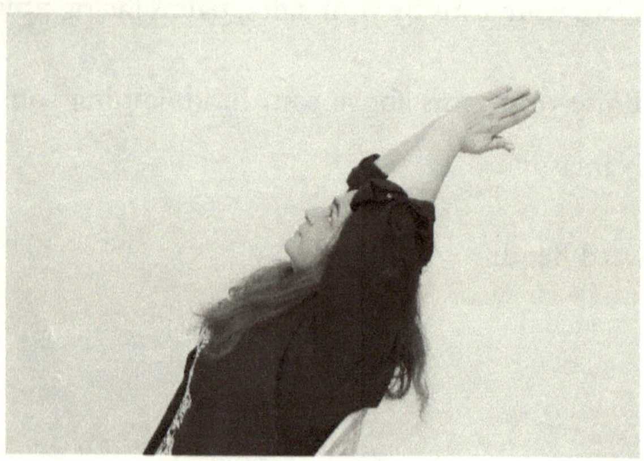

Return to an upright position, then stretch backward with your arms still in Namaste, keeping your upper arms touching your ears.

Sideward Stretch:

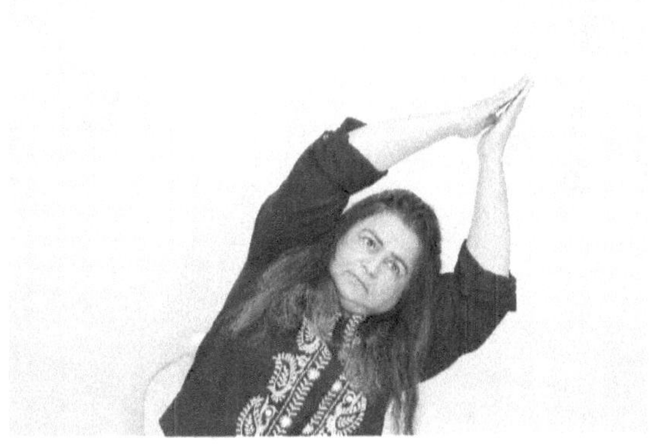

Return to the centre and tilt towards your right side, then to your left, keeping your elbows straight and upper arms touching your ears.

Twist:

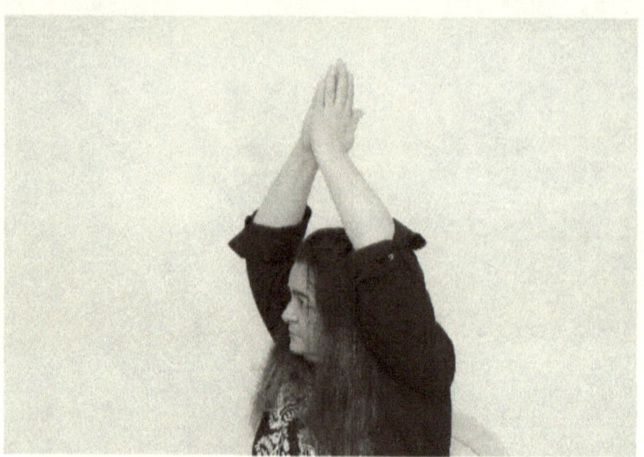

With your elbows straight, twist your torso to the right from your waist.

Repeat the twist to the left side.

Upward Stretch:

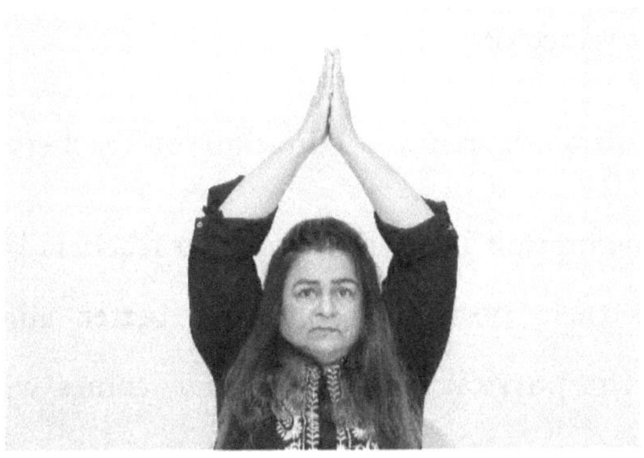

Return to the centre and stretch your arms upward.

Release the Asana:

Turn your palms outward and slowly bring your arms down.

Essentials:

Maintain each position for a count of 5 breaths.

Keep your movements smooth and controlled, focusing on your breath.

By practicing Sitting Parvatasana, you can enhance spinal flexibility, improve posture, and promote overall well-being, even while seated on a chair.

5. Postural Awareness Meditation for Teachers

This meditation is designed to help teachers become more aware of their posture, promoting better alignment and reducing the physical strain that often comes with teaching. Practicing postural awareness can lead to improved comfort, focus, and overall well-being.

Preparation:

- Find a quiet space where you won't be disturbed.

- Sit comfortably in a chair with your feet flat on the floor, or if you prefer, sit cross-legged on a cushion.

- Ensure your spine is straight but not rigid, and your shoulders are relaxed.

Centering Breath:

"Let's begin by taking a few deep breaths. Inhale deeply through your nose, filling your lungs completely. Hold for a moment, and then exhale slowly through your mouth. Repeat this a few times, allowing your breath to become a bit deeper and slower with each cycle. Feel your body begin to relax with each exhale."

Grounding:

"Now, bring your attention to your feet. Feel the solid surface beneath them, providing support and stability. Imagine a gentle, supportive energy rising from the ground, entering through your feet, and spreading throughout your entire body. This connection to the ground provides stability and support."

Spine Alignment:

"Gently bring your awareness to your spine. Imagine a string gently pulling the top of your head toward the ceiling, lengthening your spine. Allow your vertebrae to stack naturally, one on top of the other. Feel the gentle curve in your lower back, the lift in your chest, and the balance of your head atop your spine. Your posture should feel effortless, with no strain or tension."

Shoulder Relaxation:

"Now, focus on your shoulders. On your next inhale, lift your shoulders up towards your ears, and as you exhale, roll them back and let them drop down. Feel the space you've created in your upper body. Let go of any tension in your neck and shoulders."

Chest and Heart Center:

"Bring your attention to your chest. Notice if you're collapsing forward or leaning back. Allow your chest to open and expand, inviting a sense of spaciousness and openness in your heart center. Imagine your heart as a glowing light, radiating warmth and calm throughout your body."

Breathing with Awareness:

"Now, bring your awareness to your breath. Notice the natural rise and fall of your chest and abdomen with each breath. Allow your breath to be soft and natural. With each inhale, imagine drawing in energy and vitality. With each exhale, release any remaining tension."

Mindfulness of Posture:

"Begin to scan your body from head to toe, noticing any areas of tension or misalignment. Gently adjust your posture as needed. Pay attention to how small adjustments can make a big difference in how you feel. If you notice any discomfort, acknowledge it without judgment and make a slight adjustment to relieve it."

Visualization:

"Imagine yourself standing at the front of your classroom, teaching with ease and confidence. Picture your body in perfect alignment, grounded and balanced. Visualize your students responding positively to your presence, feeling your calm and composed energy. Hold this image in your mind for a few moments."

Integration:

"As we near the end of this meditation, take a moment to appreciate the awareness you've cultivated. Know that you can return to this sense of alignment and ease at any time throughout your day. When you're ready, gently begin to deepen your breath. Wiggle your fingers and toes, and slowly open your eyes."

Closing:

"Take a moment to notice how you feel now compared to when you started. Carry this sense of postural awareness with you as you go about your day, teaching with greater ease and presence. Remember, taking care of your body is an important part of being an effective and compassionate teacher."

Tips for Daily Practice:

- Set reminders to check your posture throughout the day.

- Practice this meditation daily, even for just a few minutes, to build and maintain awareness.

- Incorporate gentle stretches and movements to relieve tension during breaks.

By practicing postural awareness meditation regularly, you can improve your posture, reduce physical discomfort, and enhance your overall teaching experience.

CHAPTER 4: EYE CARE

Importance of Eye Care

Continuous use of computers and other digital devices can cause digital eye strain, characterized by headaches, dry eyes, and blurred vision. Healthy eyes help maintain concentration, reducing the risk of errors and enhancing productivity.

Eye Care for Teachers

As educators, our eyes are constantly working hard, whether it's reading student work, preparing lesson plans, or navigating digital platforms. Implementing effective eye care practices is essential to maintaining our eye health and overall well-being.

Eye Exercises for Teachers

Palming: Rub your palms together to warm them, then cup them over your closed eyes without touching, holding for 25 to 30 seconds to soothe and relax the eye muscles.

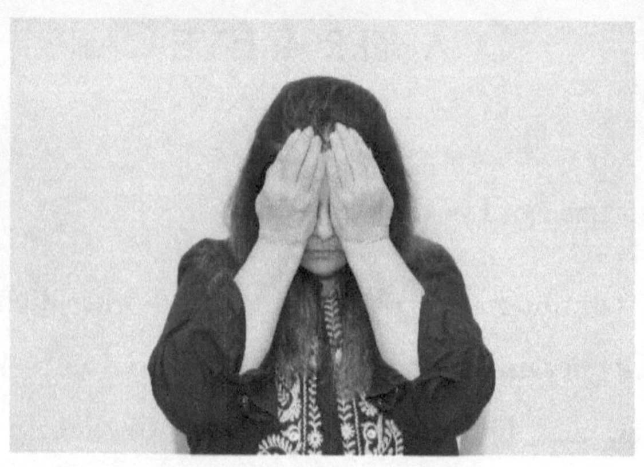

Blink often, especially when using digital devices. Blinking helps keep your eyes moist and prevents dryness.

20-20-20 rule: every 20 minutes, take a 20-second break to look at something 20 feet away. This helps reduce eye strain and gives your eyes a chance to refocus.

Ensure that your computer screen is at eye level and about an arm's length away. Adjust the brightness and contrast to comfortable levels to reduce glare. Incorporate short breaks throughout your day to rest your eyes. Use this time to stand up, stretch, and focus on distant objects.

Mudras for Eye Care

Practicing mudras can be a powerful way to support and enhance eye health. These simple hand gestures, used in conjunction with meditation and breathing exercises, can help alleviate eye strain, improve focus, and promote relaxation. Here are some effective mudras for eye care:

1. Hakini Mudra

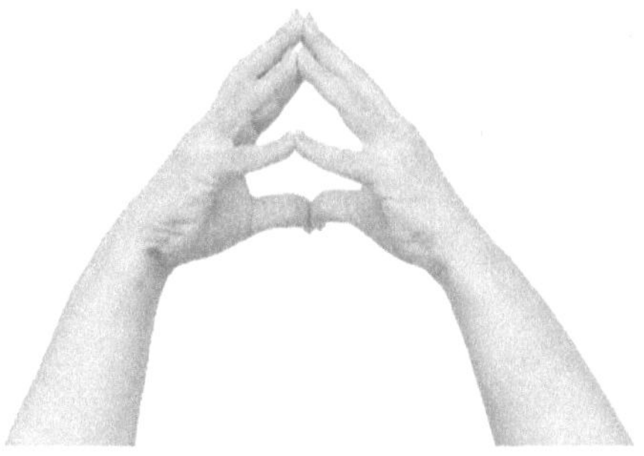

Hakini Mudra, named after the goddess Hakini, is known for its profound impact on enhancing brain power and eye health. By improving the synchronization between the brain's hemispheres, this mudra enhances eye coordination and focus, which can prevent eye strain and fatigue—a common issue for teachers who spend long hours working with books, screens, and students.

Forming the Mudra:

- Sit comfortably with your spine straight.

- Bring your hands together and touch the fingertips of both hands to each other.

- Keep the palms apart and fingers slightly bent.

- Hold this mudra at chest level.

Breathing:

- Take a deep, calming breath in through your nose.

- Exhale slowly and evenly, maintaining a sense of centeredness and balance.

Benefits:

- Stimulates the brain's cognitive functions, making it easier to focus and retain information.

- Improves coordination between the left and right hemispheres of the brain, which can benefit eye coordination and focus. This is especially useful for maintaining healthy vision and eye function.

- Calms the mind and balances brain activity alleviating anxiety and tension formed in the body, including the eyes.

Application for Teachers

For teachers, Hakini Mudra is a valuable practice to incorporate into daily routines. Here are some practical applications:

- Integrate Hakini Mudra into your daily routine to prepare your mind for the day ahead.

- Practice Hakini Mudra during short breaks to refresh your mind and maintain concentration.

- End your day with Hakini Mudra to release any accumulated stress and promote relaxation, ensuring a restful evening.

By integrating Hakini Mudra into your daily practice, you can enhance your mental and visual acuity, manage stress effectively, and create a more balanced and focused teaching environment.

2. Shambhavi Mudra

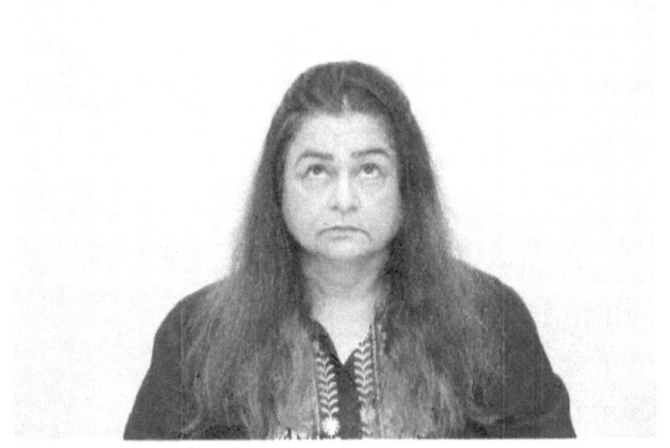

Introduction:

Shambhavi Mudra, often referred to as the "eyebrow center gazing gesture," is a powerful practice that focuses on enhancing inner awareness and concentration. By directing your gaze toward the space between the eyebrows, this mudra activates the third eye chakra, promoting mental clarity and spiritual insight. Shambhavi Mudra is particularly beneficial for teachers as it helps in maintaining focus, reducing stress, and improving overall mental well-being.

Forming the Mudra:

- Sit comfortably with your spine erect and shoulders relaxed.

- Place your hands on your knees in a comfortable position.

- Focus your eyes on a point between your eyebrows, without straining.

- Keep your gaze steady and relaxed while maintaining a calm and even breath.

Breathing:

- Take a deep, calming breath in through your nose.

- Exhale slowly and evenly, maintaining a steady, soft gaze at the eyebrow center.

Benefits:

- Improves focus and concentration.

- Reduces eye strain and fatigue.

- Calms the mind and promotes inner peace.

Application for Teachers:

For teachers, Shambhavi Mudra is a valuable practice to incorporate into daily routines. Here are some practical applications:

- Integrate into your daily routine to prepare your mind for the day ahead.

- Practice during short breaks to refresh your mind and maintain concentration.

- End your day with to release any accumulated stress and promote relaxation, ensuring a restful evening.

By integrating Shambhavi Mudra into your daily practice, you can enhance your mental clarity, manage stress effectively, and create a more balanced and focused teaching environment.

3. Varun Mudra

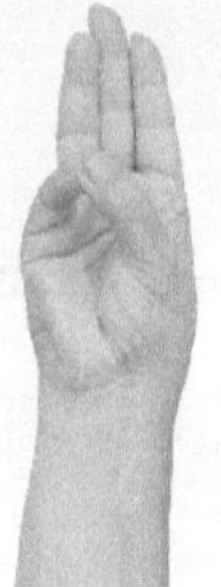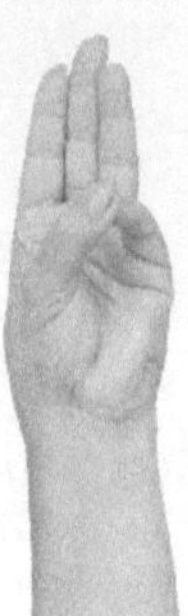

Introduction:

Varun Mudra, also known as the "water gesture," is associated with the element of water and is known for its hydrating and balancing effects. This mudra is particularly effective for maintaining eye health and preventing dryness and strain.

Forming the Mudra:

- Sit comfortably with your spine straight.

- Touch the tip of your little finger (the water element) to the tip of your thumb.

- Keep the other fingers extended and relaxed.

- Hold this mudra with both hands, resting them on your thighs or knees.

Breathing:

- Take a deep, calming breath in through your nose.

- Exhale slowly and evenly, maintaining a sense of relaxation and balance.

Benefits:

- Enhances hydration and fluid balance in the body, which is essential for eye health and preventing dryness.

- Promotes eye comfort and reduces strain, making it easier to work for long periods without discomfort.

- Calms the mind and alleviates tension, contributing to overall relaxation and well-being.

Application for Teachers:

For teachers, Varun Mudra is a valuable practice to incorporate into daily routines. Here are some practical applications:

- Start your day with Varun Mudra to hydrate your eyes and prepare for visual tasks ahead.

- During breaks, practice Varun Mudra to refresh your eyes and reduce strain.

- End your day with Varun Mudra to release any accumulated eye strain and promote relaxation, ensuring a restful evening.

By integrating Varun Mudra into your daily practice, you can maintain optimal eye health, manage stress effectively, and create a more balanced and focused teaching environment.

4. Samana Mudra (Mudra for Better Eyesight)

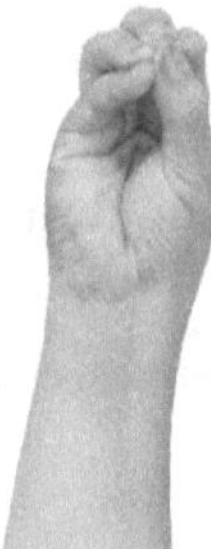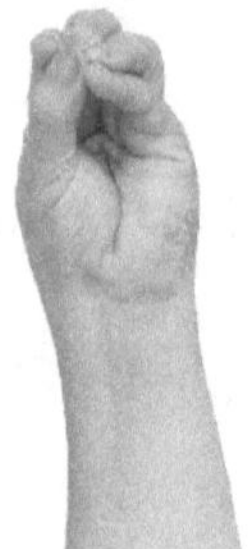

Introduction:

Samana Mudra, also known as the Mudra for Better Eyesight, is a hand gesture that helps improve vision and eye health. This mudra balances the elements in the body, promoting better blood circulation and energy flow to the eyes.

Forming the Mudra:

- Sit in a comfortable position, either on a chair with your feet flat on the ground or on the floor in a cross-legged position.

- Keep your spine straight, shoulders relaxed, and hands resting on your knees or in your lap.

- Bring the tips of your thumb, index finger, middle finger, ring finger, and little finger together to form the mudra.

Breathing:

- Inhale deeply through your nose, feeling the expansion in your chest and abdomen.

- Exhale slowly through your nose, releasing any tension while maintaining the mudra.

- Maintain a calm and rhythmic breathing pattern throughout the practice.

Benefits:

- Improves vision and overall eye health by enhancing blood circulation and energy flow to the eyes.

- Reduces eye strain and fatigue, especially from prolonged screen time or reading.

- Enhances mental clarity and focus, aiding in better concentration.

- Promotes a sense of calm and relaxation, reducing stress and tension.

Applications for Teachers:

- Incorporate Samana Mudra into your daily routine to improve and maintain eye health.

- Use it during breaks to relieve eye strain and refresh your vision.

- Practice it after prolonged periods of screen time or reading to reduce eye fatigue.

- Include it in your mindfulness or meditation sessions to enhance mental clarity and promote a sense of calm.

By regularly practicing Samana Mudra, teachers can experience improved eyesight, reduced eye strain, and enhanced mental clarity, contributing to a more effective and comfortable teaching environment.

5. Trataka Meditation for Teachers

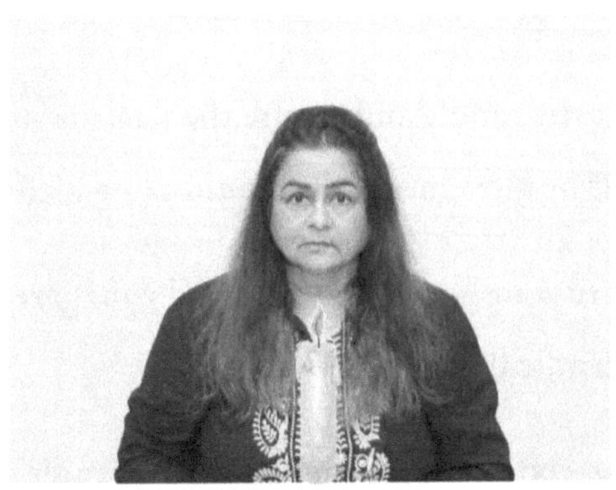

Tratak Kriya, also known as 'Yogic Gazing,' is an ancient meditation practice designed to improve eyesight. This technique involves fixing your gaze on an object until the image is imprinted in your mind when you close your eyes. It helps cleanse and rest your eyes. While Tratak is traditionally practiced with a diya or candle, it can also be performed by focusing on any object such as an idol, symbol, or even a dot on the wall.

Preparation:

- Find a quiet, dimly lit room where you won't be disturbed.

- Place a candle at eye level, about 12 to 18 inches or arm length away.

- Sit straight and still in a comfortable cross-legged position or if needed on a chair.

- Light the candle and ensure the flame is steady, free from drafts or movements that could cause it to flicker.

- Ensure your head is centered and your gaze is at level with the candle flame.

- Focus your gaze on the tip of the candle flame without blinking. Keep your eyes relaxed and your breath steady.

- Maintain a soft and steady gaze, avoiding any strain or discomfort.

- If the mind begins to wander, gently bring it back to the practice.

- After a minute or two, when the eyes become tired or begin to water, close them gently and visualize the flame between your eyebrows.

- Focus on the afterimage of the flame till it begins to fade.

- When the image starts to fade, gently cup or palm your eyes, then slowly open them.

- After a few minutes, slowly bring your awareness back to your surroundings.

- Open your eyes gently and take a few deep breaths before resuming your activities.

Benefits of Tratak:

- Activates brain cells, promoting better blood circulation and strengthening of eye muscles.

- Purifies and strengthens eye muscles by focusing on a point.

- Corrects short-sightedness.

- Helps alleviate the strain caused by prolonged screen time and reading, promoting better eye health.

- Enhances focus and attention, making it easier to manage classroom activities and student interactions.

- Helps alleviate sleep-related issues such as headaches and insomnia.

Tips for Effective Practice:

- Practice daily for 2-5 minutes, depending on individual comfort.

- Keep your eyes and face relaxed throughout the practice to avoid strain.

- Palming or cupping the eyes is mandatory after the practice of Trataka to relax the strain on the eyes

- May be performed at any time, but the best time is at dawn or dusk on empty stomach.

- Combine Trataka with mindful breathing to deepen the meditative experience and enhance relaxation.

Cautions:

- Not to be practised by those with severe mental disorder or epilepsy problem.

- Not recommended for those with serious eye disorders, the early symptoms of cataract glaucoma, or high myopia.

- People with severe myopia should keep their glasses on while practicing Trataka on a flame.

- The room should be neither too bright nor too dark.

By incorporating Trataka meditation into your daily routine, you can improve your concentration, reduce eye strain, balance the nervous system, develop good concentration and strong willpower, making it a valuable practice for all the teachers.

Drink enough water to keep your eyes and body hydrated.

Remember, taking care of your eyes is an investment in your long-term health and effectiveness as a teacher.

Incorporating Mudras into Your Routine

To gain the most benefit from these mudras, practice them regularly, ideally for 5 to 15 minutes each day. You can integrate them into your meditation or yoga routine, or use them during breaks to relieve eye strain. Remember to keep your breath steady and relaxed while practicing these mudras, as this enhances their effectiveness.

By incorporating these mudras into your daily routine, you can support your eye health, reduce strain, and enhance overall well-being. Taking a few moments each day to care for your eyes can have a significant impact on your comfort and productivity as a teacher.

CHAPTER 5: THROAT AND VOICE CARE

Voice, Hearing, and Throat Problems in Teachers

Voice Problems

Teachers often lose their voices after a fun day, event rehearsal, playground duty, or regular classroom activities. Research shows teachers are 3-5 times more likely to have voice problems and 4 times more likely to need treatment for vocal nodules than the general population. Teaching relies on effective communication, and speaking in loud, dynamic environments causes constant vocal strain. Understanding these issues and taking proactive measures is essential for maintaining vocal health and overall well-being.

Voice-Related Issues for Teachers

Continuous vocal strain can lead to:

- Prolonged speaking at high volumes causes strain, especially in noisy classrooms.

- Overusing vocal cords can lead to hoarseness or temporary voice loss.

- Excessive talking or yelling can inflame the larynx, causing a sore throat, and difficulty in speaking.

Example: A primary school teacher who spends six hours a day speaking loudly to manage an active classroom may experience chronic hoarseness and vocal fatigue by the end of the week.

Voice Care Tips for Teachers

As teachers, it's essential to care for your voice, a crucial tool for teaching and communication. Here are some tips to help you preserve your voice:

- Stay hydrated and avoid vocal extremes like shouting and whispering. Speak at a normal volume to reduce voice stress.

- Incorporate vocal rest into your routine. Alternate between activities that require heavy vocal use and those that don't. Group work can provide breaks.

- Avoid Throat Clearing as it can damage your vocal cords. Sip water and swallow hard instead.

- Use Non-Vocal Attention Grabbers like clapping rhythms, hand signals, music, whistles, or bells to get students' attention.

- Educate students on appropriate voice levels and establish quiet times to reduce the need to raise your voice.

By following these tips, you can protect your voice and ensure it remains strong and effective in your teaching toolkit.

1. Udan Mudra (Gesture of Uplifting Energy)

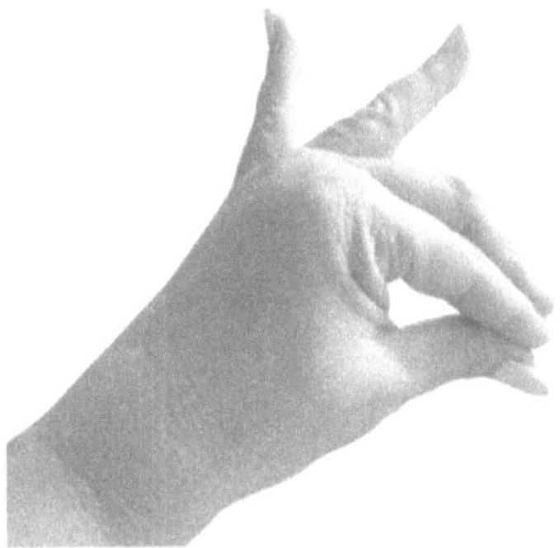

Udan Mudra, also known as the Gesture of Uplifting Energy, is a powerful mudra used in yoga and meditation to promote vitality and energy. It involves combining specific fingers to create a flow of energy that uplifts the spirit and enhances overall well-being.

Forming the Mudra:

- Sit or stand comfortably with your back straight and shoulders relaxed.

- Place your hands on your thighs or knees with palms facing upward.

- Touch the tips of your index and middle fingers to the tip of your thumb.

- Extend the ring and little fingers straight out.

- Keep the mudra steady and your hands relaxed.

Breathing:

- Take a deep, energizing breath in through your nose.

- Exhale slowly and evenly, feeling a sense of upliftment and vitality.

- Maintain a steady and rhythmic breathing pattern throughout the practice.

Benefits:

- Enhances energy levels and vitality.

- Promotes a sense of upliftment and positivity.

- Improves concentration and mental clarity.

- Supports emotional balance and reduces stress.

Applications for Teachers:

- Integrate Udan Mudra into your daily routine to boost energy and positivity.

- Use this mudra before starting your classes to enhance focus and set a positive tone.

- Practice Udan Mudra during short breaks to alleviate stress and rejuvenate your energy.

By regularly practicing Udan Mudra, teachers can experience increased energy, reduced stress, and a greater sense of positivity, contributing to a more effective and harmonious teaching environment.

2. Shankh Mudra (Conch Shell Gesture)

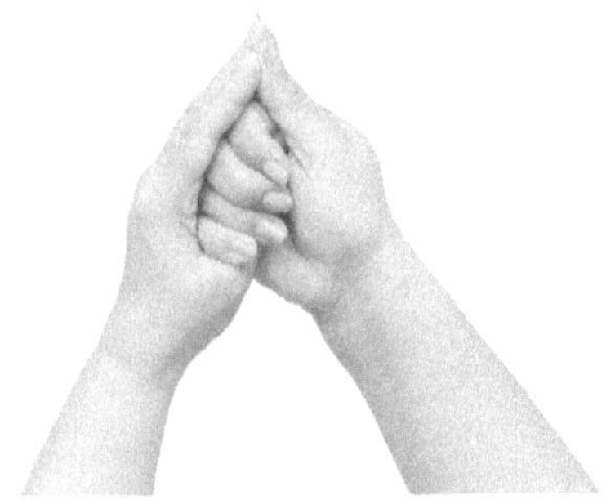

Shankh Mudra, also known as the Conch Shell Gesture, is a significant mudra in yoga and meditation symbolizing the sacred sound of Om. It is used to balance the throat chakra and improve communication and clarity.

Forming the Mudra:

- Sit comfortably with your back straight and shoulders relaxed.

- Hold your left thumb with the fingers of your right hand.

- Touch the tip of your right thumb to the tip of your left middle finger.

- Wrap the other fingers of your left hand around your right thumb.

- Hold the mudra at chest level.

Breathing:

- Take a deep, calming breath in through your nose.

- Exhale slowly and evenly, maintaining a sense of centeredness and clarity.

- Maintain a steady and rhythmic breathing pattern throughout the practice.

Benefits:

- Balances the throat chakra, enhancing communication and self-expression.

- Reduces stress and promotes a sense of calm.

- Improves respiratory function and clarity of thought.

- Supports emotional and mental balance, aiding in overall well-being.

Applications for Teachers:

- Integrate Shankh Mudra into your daily routine to enhance communication and clarity.

- Use this mudra before starting your classes to center yourself and set a positive tone.

- Practice Shankh Mudra during short breaks to alleviate stress and regain focus.

By regularly practicing Shankh Mudra, teachers can experience improved communication, reduced stress, and a greater sense of balance, contributing to a more effective and harmonious teaching environment.

3. Vishuddha Mudra (Purification Gesture)

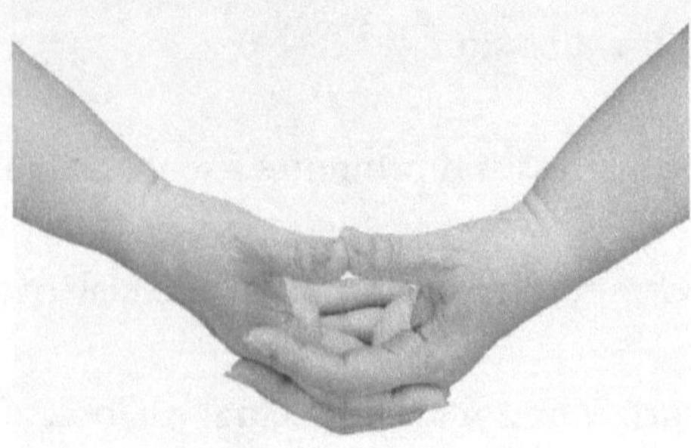

Vishuddha Mudra, also known as the Purification Gesture, is a powerful mudra used in yoga to balance the throat chakra, enhancing communication and clarity.

Forming the Mudra:

- Sit comfortably with your back straight and shoulders relaxed.

- Interlace the fingers of both hands, except the thumbs, which should be extended and touching at the tips.

- Hold the mudra at your throat level, with the thumbs pointing upwards.

Breathing:

- Take a deep, calming breath in through your nose.

- Exhale slowly and evenly, maintaining a sense of centeredness and clarity.

- Maintain a steady and rhythmic breathing pattern throughout the practice.

Benefits:

- Balances the throat chakra, improving communication and self-expression.

- Reduces stress and promotes a sense of calm.

- Enhances clarity of thought and focus.

- Supports emotional and mental balance, aiding in overall well-being.

Applications for Teachers:

- Integrate Vishuddha Mudra into your daily routine to enhance communication and clarity.

- Use this mudra before starting your classes to center yourself and set a positive tone.

- Practice Vishuddha Mudra during short breaks to alleviate stress and regain focus.

By regularly practicing Vishuddha Mudra, teachers can experience improved communication, reduced stress, and a greater sense of balance, contributing to a more effective and harmonious teaching environment.

4. Simha Mudra (Lion Gesture)

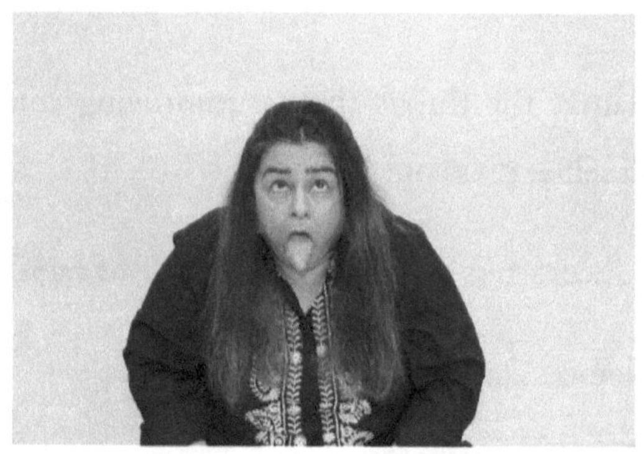

Simha Mudra, also known as the Lion Gesture, is a powerful mudra used in yoga to release tension, improve vocal strength, and stimulate energy. It mimics a lion's roar, helping to relieve stress and enhance confidence.

Forming the Mudra:

- Sit comfortably with your back straight and shoulders relaxed, preferably in a kneeling position (Vajrasana).

- Place your hands on your knees, spreading your fingers wide.

- Inhale deeply through your nose.

- As you exhale, open your mouth wide, stretch your tongue out as far as possible, and produce a sound from your throat like a roaring lion.

Breathing:

- Take a deep, energizing breath in through your nose.

- Exhale forcefully while making the roaring sound, releasing all tension.

- Maintain a steady and rhythmic breathing pattern throughout the practice.

Benefits:

- Releases tension and stress, particularly in the face and throat.

- Enhances vocal strength and clarity.

- Stimulates energy and boosts confidence.

- Supports emotional release and overall well-being.

Applications for Teachers:

- Integrate Simha Mudra into your daily routine to release tension and boost confidence.

- Use this mudra before starting your classes to energize yourself and set a positive tone.

- Practice Simha Mudra during short breaks to alleviate stress and rejuvenate your energy.

By regularly practicing Simha Mudra, teachers can experience reduced stress, improved vocal strength, and increased confidence, contributing to a more effective and harmonious teaching environment.

5. Bhramari Pranayama (Humming Bee Breath)

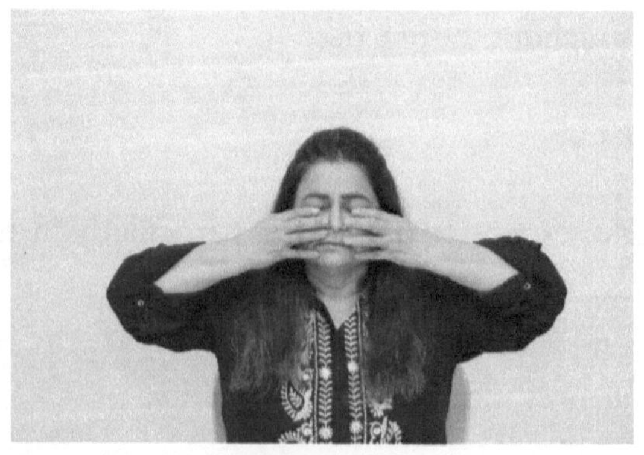

Pranayama is a yogic practice that involves breath control techniques to enhance physical and mental well-being. Bhramari Pranayama, is known for its calming and soothing effects on the mind and body. It involves producing a humming sound during exhalation, which resonates in the head and helps quiet the mind.

Preparation:

- Find a quiet and comfortable place to sit, either on the floor in a cross-legged position or on a chair with your feet flat on the ground.

- Get ready in Shanmukhi Mudra, by sitting comfortably with your back straight and shoulders relaxed. Raise your hands to your face and use your thumbs to gently close your ears, index fingers lightly over your closed eyelids, middle fingers on the sides of your nose, ring fingers above your lips, and little fingers below your lips.

Breathing Pattern:

- Take a deep breath in through your nose, filling your lungs completely.

- As you exhale slowly and steadily, make a steady humming sound like that of a bee.

- Focus on feeling the vibration of the sound resonating in your head and throughout your body.

Duration: Start with 5 rounds of Bhramari Pranayama, gradually increasing to 10 rounds. Practice daily for optimal benefits.

Benefits of Bhramari Pranayama

- Enhances the quality and depth of your voice tone, beneficial for teachers who speak extensively in classrooms.

- Exercises the vocal cords without strain, promoting vocal health and longevity.

- Acts as a gentle massage for throat muscles, promoting relaxation and warmth.

- Improves breath control, aiding in clear and effective speech delivery for teachers.

Applications for Teachers

1. Teachers can benefit from Bhramari Pranayama to maintain vocal health, improve tone, and reduce strain from extensive speaking in classrooms.

2. Regular practice helps teachers manage stress and maintain emotional balance, crucial for a positive teaching environment.

3. Improved breath control and vocal clarity from Bhramari Pranayama can enhance teachers' presence and effectiveness in delivering lessons.

4. Incorporating into daily routines help warm up vocal cords, relax throat muscles, and prepare for a day of teaching.

5. Beyond the classroom, teachers can use Bhramari Pranayama to unwind, relax, and rejuvenate, fostering overall well-being.

By integrating Bhramari Pranayama into their daily practice, teachers can enhance their vocal performance, manage stress effectively, and create a more conducive learning environment for their students.

Conclusion

Teachers' voices, hearing, and throat health are crucial for their professional effectiveness and overall well-being. By understanding these common issues and taking proactive measures, teachers can protect their vocal and auditory health, ensuring a long and healthy career in education.

CHAPTER 6: HEARING

Hearing Problems in Teachers

Teachers often experience hearing problems due to the noisy environments in which they work. Classrooms, playgrounds, and school assemblies can be loud and chaotic, putting significant strain on teachers' auditory systems. Over time, this constant exposure to high noise levels can lead to hearing fatigue, tinnitus, and even hearing loss.

- Prolonged exposure to noisy classrooms can lead to gradual hearing loss.

- Continuous loud sounds can cause persistent ringing or buzzing in the ears.

- Poor classroom acoustics and frequent headphone use can lead to ear infections.

Preventive Measures

Classroom Management: Implement classroom noise management strategies, such as using non-verbal signals for attention, establishing quiet times, and encouraging students to speak at a reasonable volume.

Acoustic Modifications: Improve classroom acoustics with sound-absorbing materials like carpets, curtains, and wall panels to reduce noise levels and create a more auditory-friendly environment.

Quiet Time: Dedicate time each day to sit in a quiet space, allowing your ears to rest and recover from auditory strain. This can help prevent hearing fatigue and maintain auditory health.

1. Shunya Mudra (Mudra of Emptiness)

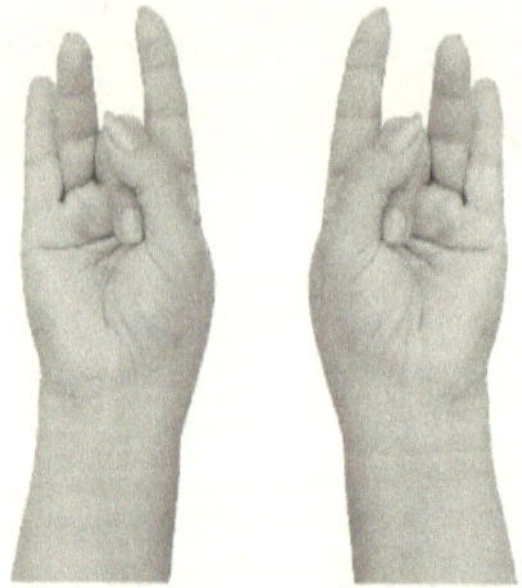

Introduction:

Shunya Mudra, also known as the Mudra of Emptiness, is a hand gesture practiced in yoga and Ayurveda to balance the element of space (Akasha) in the body. This mudra is particularly beneficial for addressing ear-related issues and enhancing auditory functions. Shunya Mudra is derived from the Sanskrit word "Shunya," which means "zero" or "emptiness," symbolizing the reduction of the space element in the body.

Forming the Mudra:

- Sit comfortably with your back straight and shoulders relaxed.

- Bend your middle finger and place its tip at the base of your thumb.

- Gently press your thumb over the bent middle finger.

- Keep the other fingers extended and relaxed.

Breathing:

- Take a deep, calming breath in through your nose.

- Exhale slowly and evenly, feeling a sense of peace and relaxation.

- Maintain a steady and rhythmic breathing pattern throughout the practice.

Benefits:

- Alleviates ear problems such as earaches and tinnitus.

- Promotes a sense of inner peace and calm.

- Enhances concentration and mental clarity.

- Supports emotional and mental balance, aiding in overall well-being.

Applications for Teachers:

- Integrate Shunya Mudra into your daily routine to promote calmness and clarity.

- Use this mudra before starting your classes to center yourself and set a positive tone.

- Practice Shunya Mudra during short breaks to alleviate stress and regain focus.

By regularly practicing Shunya Mudra, teachers can experience reduced stress, improved mental clarity, and a greater sense of balance, contributing to a more effective and harmonious teaching environment.

2. Akash Mudra (Space Mudra)

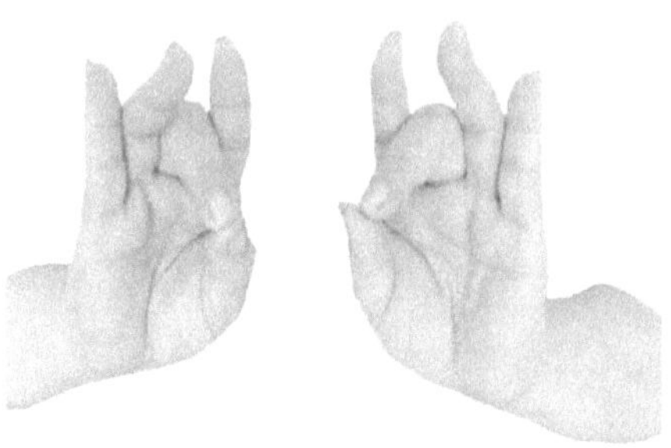

Akash Mudra, also known as the Gesture of the Sky, is a significant mudra in yoga and meditation that helps to enhance mental clarity and spiritual awareness by balancing the space element within the body.

Forming the Mudra:

- Sit comfortably with your back straight and shoulders relaxed.

- Touch the tip of your middle finger to the tip of your thumb.

- Keep the other three fingers extended and relaxed.

- Rest your hands on your knees with palms facing upward.

Breathing:

- Take a deep, calming breath in through your nose.

- Exhale slowly and evenly, maintaining a sense of openness and expansiveness.

- Maintain a steady and rhythmic breathing pattern throughout the practice.

Benefits:

- Enhances mental clarity and focus.

- Promotes a sense of openness and expansiveness.

- Reduces feelings of heaviness and promotes lightness in the body.

- Supports spiritual awareness and emotional balance, aiding in overall well-being.

Applications for Teachers:

- Integrate Akash Mudra into your daily routine to enhance mental clarity and focus.

- Use this mudra before starting your classes to center yourself and set a positive tone.

- Practice Akash Mudra during short breaks to alleviate stress and regain a sense of openness and balance.

By regularly practicing Akash Mudra, teachers can enhance auditory function, reduce ear-related issues, and promote overall well-being.

3. Greeva Chalan (Neck Movements)

With age, decreased blood supply to the brain and inner ear can lead to cervical spondylosis, which often results in a gradual loss of hearing. Fortunately, regular cervical and shoulder exercises can help alleviate tension and maintain neck health. Here are three beneficial exercises:

1. Lift your head upward as far as comfortable, stretching your neck backward.

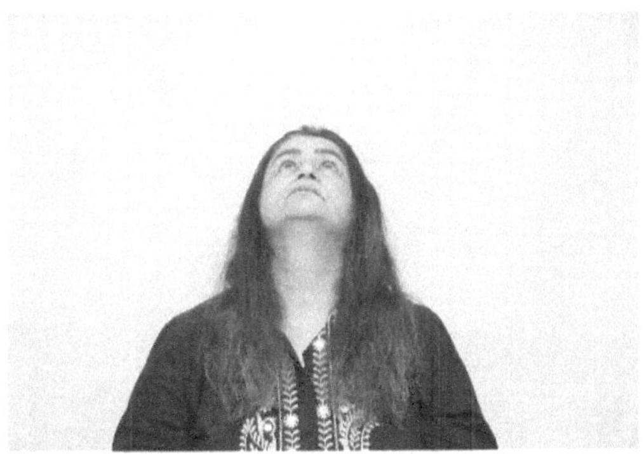

2. Without turning or rotating your head, gently tilt your head to the right, attempting to touch your right ear to your right shoulder. Repeat the movement on the left side, bringing your left ear towards your left shoulder.

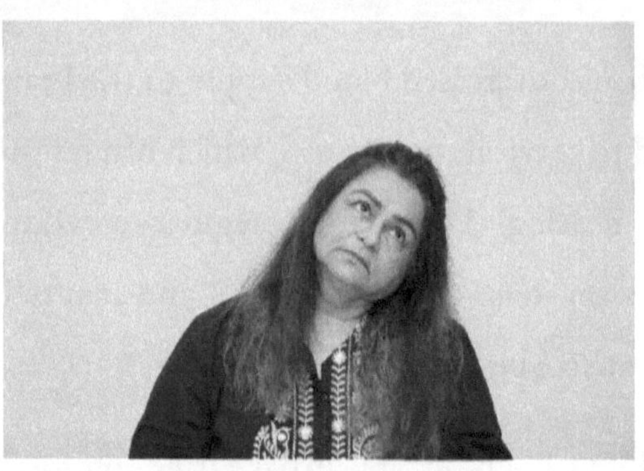

3. Start by rotating your head to the right. Return to the neutral position, then rotate your head to the left.

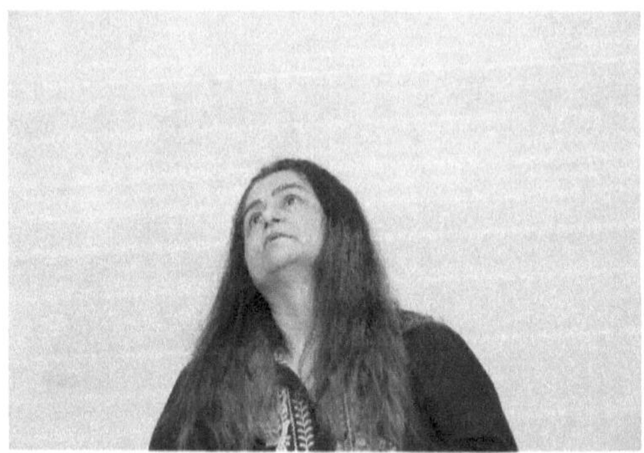

Ensure smooth and controlled movements to avoid strain. Regular practice of these exercises can help improve blood circulation, reduce tension, and support overall neck health.

4. Skandh Chalan (Rotating the Shoulders)

Skandh Chalan, or Rotating the Shoulders, is an effective exercise that enhances flexibility and improves posture. This practice draws awareness to the upper body and spine, helping to alleviate postural issues such as hunching. Additionally, it can indirectly benefit hearing by improving blood circulation and reducing tension around the neck and shoulders, which can affect ear health.

Instructions:

Starting Position:

- Sit on the chair with your legs crossed or placing them on the floor.

- Place your right hand on your right knee and your left hand on your left knee.

Shoulder Rotation:

- Rotate your right shoulder in a circular motion: up, forward, down, and back.

- Simultaneously, rotate your left shoulder in the opposite direction: down, back, up, and forward.

- Ensure that when one shoulder is up, the other is down.

- Perform 4 rotations in one direction.

- Then, reverse the rotation and perform 4 more rotations in the opposite direction.

Ensure smooth and controlled movements to avoid strain. Regular practice of these exercises can help improve posture, increase flexibility, and reduce shoulder tension. Improved circulation and reduced tension around the neck and shoulders can alleviate pressure on the nerves and blood vessels linked to the ears, potentially benefiting hearing health.

5. Ear Massage for Better Hearing

Ear massage is an effective technique to improve circulation and stimulate the auditory nerves, potentially enhancing hearing capabilities. Here are detailed steps for performing an ear massage:

1. Ear Lobe Massage

- Gently grasp your ear lobes between your thumb and index finger.

- Gently pull your ear lobes downward and then upward, applying light pressure.

- Massage the lobes in small circular motions for about 30 seconds.

2. Outer Ear Massage

- Use your fingers to gently massage the outer part of your ear in circular motions.

- Continue this circular massage for about 30 seconds, gradually increasing pressure as comfortable.

3. Helix Massage

- Using your thumb and index finger, gently pinch the upper part of your ear, known as the helix.

- Slowly move your fingers along the helix from the top of your ear down to the earlobe.

- Repeat this motion several times, applying gentle pressure.

4. Tug(pull) and Release

- Grasp the upper part of your ears with your thumb and index finger.

- Gently tug your ears upward, hold for a few seconds, and then release.

- Next, grasp the middle part of your ears and gently tug outward, hold, and release.

- Finally, grasp the earlobes and gently tug downward, hold, and release.

5. Press and Release

- Using the palms of your hands, cover your ears completely and gently press.

- Quickly remove your hands to create a slight vacuum effect, stimulating the ears.

- Repeat this several times for added stimulation.

Benefits of Ear Massage:

- Enhances blood flow to the ears, which can help maintain ear health and function.

- Activates the auditory nerves, potentially improving hearing clarity.

- Relieves tension around the ears and temples, promoting relaxation.

- Maintains and even improves auditory function over time.

Integrating ear massage into your daily routine can contribute to better ear health and potentially enhance hearing capabilities. Regular practice can also serve as a soothing, stress-relieving activity.

Chapter 7: Heart Health

The Importance of Heart Health for Teachers

Teachers dedicate their lives to educating and inspiring students, often putting their own well-being on the backburner. Maintaining heart health is crucial for teachers as it impacts their personal well-being, professional performance, and overall quality of life. Prioritizing cardiovascular health can lead to improved energy, mood, and effectiveness in the classroom.

Why Heart Health is Important for Teachers

- A healthy heart ensures good circulation, delivering oxygen and nutrients throughout the body, supporting sustained energy levels for active teaching.

- Proper blood flow supports cognitive abilities such as concentration, memory, and decision-making, crucial for effective teaching.

- Maintaining heart health helps manage stress, leading to improved emotional stability and resilience.

- Good cardiovascular health reduces the risk of chronic conditions like hypertension and diabetes, leading to fewer absences and a better quality of life.

- Prioritizing heart health contributes to a longer, healthier life, enhancing motivation and enthusiasm in teaching.

- Teachers who demonstrate healthy habits inspire students to adopt a healthy lifestyle, promoting overall well-being in the next generation.

Causes and Contributing Factors of Heart-Related Problems for Teachers

- Stress: Constant pressure from workload, deadlines, and student behaviour.

- Sedentary Lifestyle: Long hours of sitting while teaching or grading.

- Poor Diet: Limited time for healthy meals, leading to reliance on fast food.

- Lack of Exercise: Busy schedules leaving little time for physical activity.

- Sleep Deprivation: Grading and lesson planning cutting into rest time.

Strategies

Regular physical activity, healthy diet, stress managing, adequate sleep, hydration and avoidance of harmful habits can help prevent the problem.

Practical Tips for Teachers

- Classroom Environment: Create a calming classroom environment with plants, soothing colours, and relaxing music.

- Time Management: Prioritize tasks and set realistic goals to reduce overwhelm.

- Delegate Tasks: Whenever possible, delegate administrative tasks to reduce workload.

- Take Breaks: Schedule regular breaks throughout the day to relax and recharge.

1. Apana Mudra (Gesture of Vital Energy)

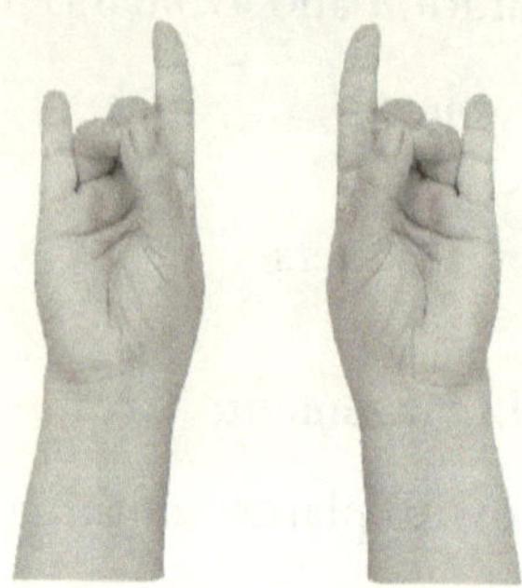

Apana Mudra, also known as the Mudra of Digestion and Elimination, is a powerful hand gesture used in yoga and meditation to promote physical and mental well-being. This mudra helps detoxify the body, improve digestion, and balance energy, which can significantly aid in managing hypertension (high blood pressure).

Forming the Mudra:

- Sit comfortably with your back straight and shoulders relaxed.

- Touch the tips of your thumb, middle finger, and ring finger together.

- Keep the index finger and little finger extended.

- Rest your hands on your knees with palms facing upward.

Breathing:

- Take a deep, calming breath in through your nose.

- Exhale slowly and evenly, feeling a sense of release and detoxification.

- Maintain a steady and rhythmic breathing pattern throughout the practice.

Benefits:

- Helps detoxify and purify the body.

- Balances the body's energies, promoting overall well-being.

- Supports digestive health and alleviates constipation.

- Enhances mental clarity and emotional stability.

Applications for Teachers:

- Integrate Apana Mudra into your daily routine to support detoxification and energy balance.

- Use this mudra before starting your classes to center yourself and set a positive tone.

- Practice Apana Mudra during short breaks to alleviate stress and regain focus.

For teachers, who often face high levels of stress and long hours, practicing Apana Mudra can be a valuable tool for maintaining heart health and overall wellness.

2. Apana Vayu Mudra (Gesture of the Heart)

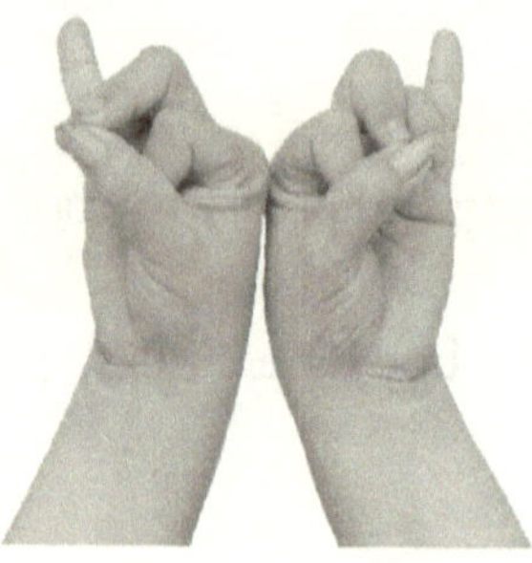

Apana Vayu Mudra, also known as the Heart Mudra or Mrita Sanjeevani Mudra, is a powerful hand gesture to support heart health. This mudra is particularly effective in balancing the body's energy and promoting cardiovascular well-being. For teachers, who often deal with high stress and long hours, practicing Apana Vayu Mudra can be a valuable tool for maintaining a healthy heart and reducing hypertension.

Forming the Mudra:

- Sit comfortably with your back straight and shoulders relaxed.

- Touch the tips of your thumb, middle finger, and ring finger together.

- Bend your index finger to touch the base of your thumb.

- Keep the little finger extended.

- Rest your hands on your knees with palms facing upward.

Breathing:

- Take a deep, calming breath in through your nose.

- Exhale slowly and evenly, feeling a sense of calm and balance.

- Maintain a steady and rhythmic breathing pattern throughout the practice.

Benefits:

- Calms the heart and mind, reducing anxiety and stress.

- Improves circulation and cardiovascular health.

- Enhances overall emotional stability.

- Promotes a sense of inner peace and well-being.

Applications for Teachers:

- Integrate Apana Vayu Mudra into your daily routine to promote heart health and emotional stability.

- Use this mudra before starting your classes to center yourself and set a positive tone.

- Practice Apana Vayu Mudra during short breaks to alleviate stress and regain focus.

By regularly practicing Apana Vayu Mudra, teachers can experience improved heart health, reduced stress, and a greater sense of balance, contributing to a more effective and harmonious teaching environment.

3. Surya Mudra (Gesture of the Sun)

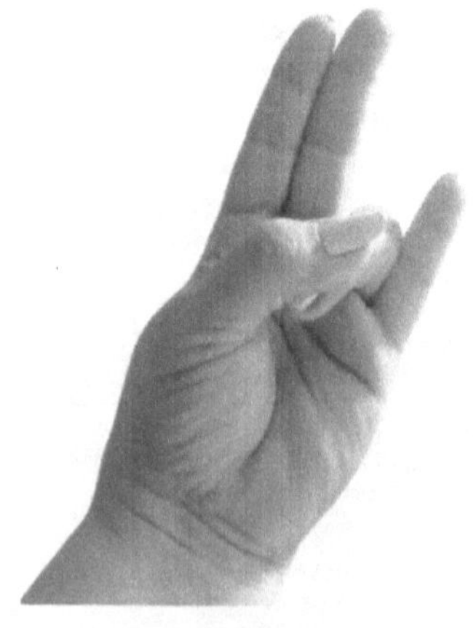

Surya Mudra, also known as the Mudra of the Sun, boosts energy, improve metabolism, and enhance overall well-being. This mudra is particularly effective in reducing high blood pressure and bad cholesterol (LDL) by promoting better digestion, improving circulation, and reducing stress.

Forming the Mudra:

- Sit comfortably with your back straight and shoulders relaxed.

- Fold your ring finger to touch the base of your thumb.

- Press the ring finger gently with your thumb.

- Keep the other fingers extended and relaxed.

- Rest your hands on your knees with palms facing upward.

Breathing:

- Take a deep, invigorating breath in through your nose.

- Exhale slowly and evenly, feeling a sense of warmth and energy.

- Maintain a steady and rhythmic breathing pattern throughout the practice.

Benefits:

- Increases energy and vitality.

- Boosts metabolism and aids in weight management.

- Improves digestion and reduces lethargy.

- Enhances overall mental clarity and focus.

Applications for Teachers:

- Integrate Surya Mudra into your daily routine to increase energy and vitality.

- Use this mudra before starting your classes to feel energized and set a positive tone.

- Practice Surya Mudra during short breaks to alleviate fatigue and regain focus.

Incorporating Surya Mudra into your daily routine can help manage high blood pressure, reduce bad cholesterol, and promote overall well-being, enhancing your ability to be an effective and healthy teacher.

4. Meditation "Finding Calm in the Classroom"

Start by finding a comfortable position, either seated or lying down. Close your eyes and take a deep breath in through your nose, filling your lungs completely. Hold for a moment, then slowly exhale through your mouth.

As you continue to breathe deeply and rhythmically, imagine a warm, golden light entering your body with each inhalation. This light represents calm and relaxation, spreading throughout your entire being. With each exhale, release any tension, stress, or worry, letting it dissolve into the air.

Visualize yourself in your classroom, but this time, it's a place of serenity and peace. The walls are adorned with calming colors, and the air is filled with a gentle, soothing fragrance. You feel a sense of control and ease.

Picture your students, each one surrounded by a gentle, glowing light. They are attentive, calm, and eager to learn. You are guiding them with a steady hand and a peaceful heart.

Take a moment to acknowledge the important role you play in their lives. Feel the gratitude they have for your dedication and care. Let this sense of appreciation fill your heart and mind.

Now, imagine a protective bubble around yourself. This bubble allows positive energy and love to flow in while keeping stress and negativity out. You are safe, you are calm, and you are in control.

As you begin to bring your awareness back to the present moment, carry with you this sense of calm and peace. Know that you can return to this place of tranquility whenever you need it.

Take a final deep breath in, hold it for a moment, and then exhale fully. When you are ready, gently open your eyes and return to your day, refreshed and centered.

Conclusion

Maintaining heart health is essential for teachers to ensure they have the energy, focus, and emotional stability needed to excel in their profession. By adopting healthy lifestyle habits and managing stress effectively, teachers can improve their cardiovascular health, enhance their overall quality of life, and set a positive example for their students. Prioritizing heart health benefits not only teachers personally but also positively impacts their professional effectiveness and well-being.

DISCLAIMER

While the practices and techniques shared in this book are based on my personal experiences and research, it is important to understand that they are not intended as a substitute for professional medical advice, diagnosis, or treatment. The information provided is meant to serve as a guide for enhancing well-being and balance in your teaching practice, but individual results may vary.

I encourage you to consult with a healthcare provider before beginning any new health practice, especially if you have any pre-existing conditions or concerns. The exercises and mudras presented here are meant to complement your overall well-being, not replace any medical or therapeutic interventions. Your safety and health are paramount, so please listen to your body and proceed with mindfulness and care.

ABOUT THE AUTHOR

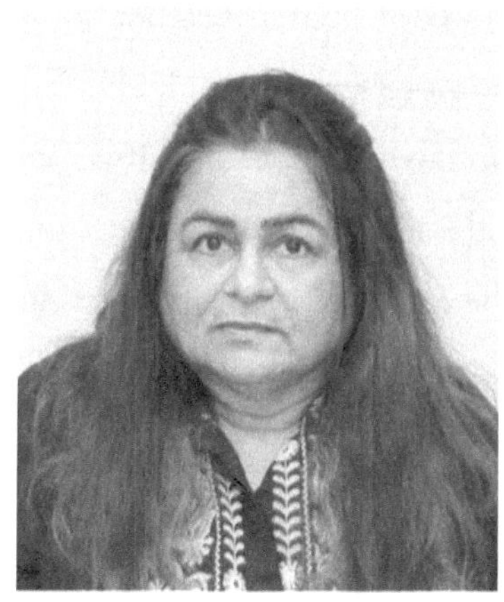

Shilpa Mehta: *A Journey of Yoga and Lifelong Learning*

Shilpa Mehta embarked on her Yoga journey in 1996, immersing herself in the true essence of Yoga at an ashram. Her practice deepened through training at esteemed institutions such as The Yoga Institute, Kaivalya Dham, Shri Ambika Yoga Kutir, and Mumbai University. During this period, she also taught Kathak dance and pre-primary classes, showcasing her versatility as an educator.

An avid reader, traveler, and YouTuber, Shilpa began sharing her Yoga expertise in 1998. Over the years, she has conducted various health camps for professionals, including doctors, executives, chartered accountants, and teachers. Originally focusing on physical platform, Shilpa now extends her teachings online, reaching a global audience.

Shilpa has also coordinated teacher training courses at The Yoga Institute for more than a decade. Holding a master's degree in philosophy and having studied positive psychology, she brings a deep intellectual and emotional understanding to her practice. Additionally, she has served as a speaker and judge at international Yoga conferences.

Currently, Shilpa teaches Yoga at Dhirubhai Ambani International School and has been dedicated to her craft for over 21 years. Her passion for Yoga not only ignites her purpose in life but also fulfills it through both practice and teaching.

May I Ask You For A Small Favor?

At the outset, I want to thank you for reading this book. You could have chosen any other book, but you took mine, and I appreciate this.

I hope you got at least a few actionable insights that will positively impact your day-to-day life.

Can I ask for 30 seconds more of your time?

I'd love it if you could leave a review of the book. That will help me grow my readership by encouraging folks to take a chance on my books.

Keeping it straight - reviews are the lifeblood of any author.

It will take less than a minute of your time but will help me reach out to more people.

If you enjoyed this book, I would greatly appreciate it if you could leave an honest review where you purchased it. I'd love to read your thoughts. Thank you for your support!